A HEALTHY GUIDE TO EATING

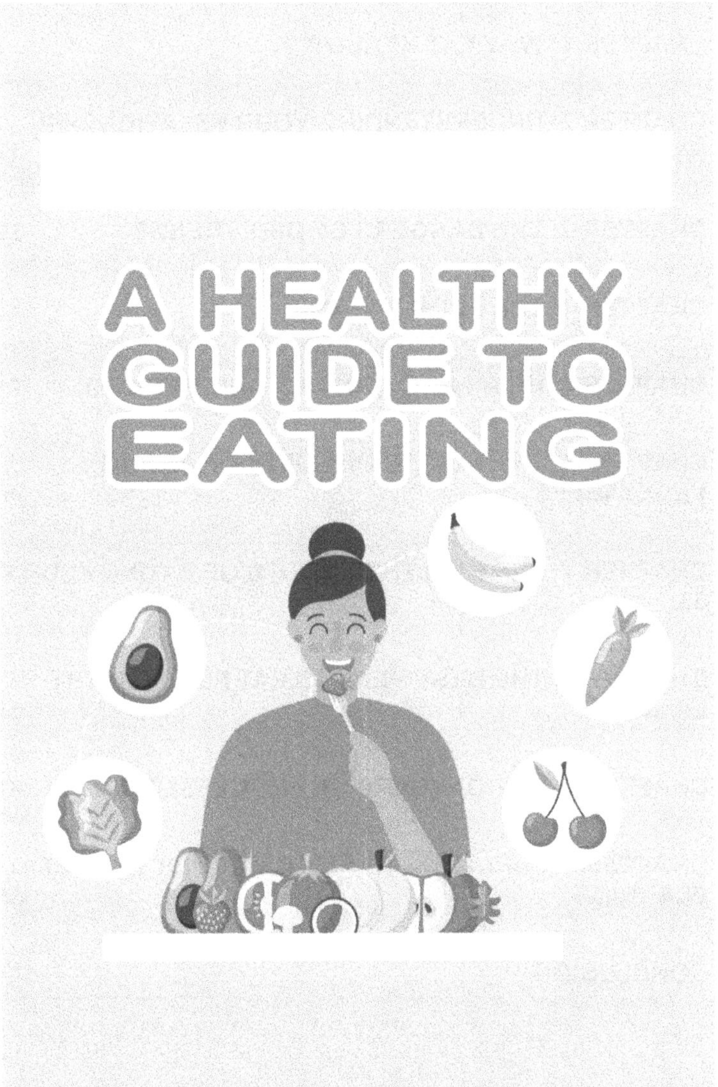

introduction

For a few reason, one of the hardest things for a human to do is to eat right. Whether that's since we have constrained get to to assets in all ranges or in case it is since we basically have as well much get to to undesirable nourishment, there are numerous reasons that eating healthy could be a challenge.

Sure, we are able eat almost anything and it'll maintain us. We'll oversee to move from one minute to the following and be able to call ourselves solid. But is it sound to subsist on a slim down of handled nourishments and sugary drinks? Just because we are lively does not cruel that we are sound. And the more seasoned we get, the more our awful propensities start to catch up with us.

It is incredibly critical to make solid eating propensities early on in life, or at slightest, as early as conceivable to anticipate any future issues from occurring. You are doing not need to wake up one day and realize that you just have had a supplement insufficiency for a long time and it is causing complications that are nearly outlandish to correct. All of us got to take more duty for what we put into our bodies, since on the off chance that we don't, it can ended up greatly perilous.

Of course, when we are older and we are ready to see back on our botches, insight into the past is 20/20. We realize that there were things that we may have done and likely should have done that we basically didn't do because we were either oblivious of the ill impacts, or simply lazy. Fair having the basic information does not fundamentally make at that point has to do something healthconscious a reality.

For the foremost portion, it takes us really being uncovered to the enduring that can happen since of awful wellbeing choices some time recently we are more cognizant of the way we treat our bodies and our wellbeing in general. When we aren't able to see the reality of the results to our activities, it can make them feel

very distant away and difficult to relate to. We may even blow them off entirely. This may be a really weakening put to discover yourself in. Particularly after you are as of now managing from the side impacts of destitute eating and a need of a sound eat less.

Everybody merits a chance to ended up the most prominent form of themselves conceivable, but in the event that we are not indeed recognizing the truth that unfortunate eating can take us right off course, even in the present minute, at that point we are eventually waving farewell to the most excellent future conceivable.
But all of this will alter. By perusing this book, you're aiming to get it the significance of eating solid and how nourishment

impacts our bodies and capacities.

Without understanding exactly why our bodies respond to nourishment the way they do, it can in some cases be troublesome to stay on track. But there are numerous ways merely can start to get it why eating sound nourishments is so important, and precisely how to start on a sound eating travel. Let's not squander any more time. We should begin eating sound today!

CHAPTER 1: WHY EAT HEALTHY?

Solid eating is critical for a part of reasons. Most of us are as of now mindful of the expanding weight scourge in North America. Typically especially true of the Joined together States in common. There's even a express for the way numerous Americans eat, which is called the Pitiful slim down.

SAD stands for standard American count calories, and it alludes to a count calories moo in vegetables, tall in fat and sugar, and missing in nourishment. Prepared nourishments are unquestionably a portion of the Pitiful eat less. These are nourishments that are effectively accessible and quick to consume and plan but have long-lasting negative wellbeing impacts.

If you are doing not need to discover yourself stout, it is for the most part considered a great thought to dodge eating such prepared nourishments and keep your center on eating entirety grains and natural products and vegetables and meat that has not been treated with hormones and other chemicals that can eventually conclusion up in your body and cause issues. Tragically, in North America, we are given a part of choices to slack off when it comes to planning meals.

We have so numerous things promptly accessible to us, and the sum of cash simply need to spend to purchase terrible nourishment is distant less at that point it is to buy great nourishment. It appears bizarre that it costs more money to purchase natural than it does to purchase nourishments that will eventually cause wellbeing issues within the long run, but that is the run the show of supply and request.

Not as it were that, but processed nourishments are mass-produced and make a colossal benefit since of their convenience. That's why, in numerous ways, and weight plague in North America isn't especially shocking. Nutrition isn't number one on the list of companies that are endeavoring to cash in on people's sluggishness in the kitchen.

However, there are many ways that eating solid is vital, and great reasons to maintain a strategic distance from handled nourishments and the standard American slim down. For case, in the event that you are doing not need to be stout, you should definitely see into the rest of this book for ways to move forward your slim down and start a more advantageous lifestyle.

Another reason to eat healthy is since you'll make yourself inclined to infections by eating undesirable nourishments and by remaining on a standard American slim down that's full of fat and sugar. Diabetes is something that can be created since of destitute eating and can regularly times be treated with sound eating.

Type II diabetes is ultimately something that can be kept up and controlled with appropriate eating habits and activated by destitute eating habits. If you need to avoid these sorts of troubles and complications, you ought to do your best to be honest around your nourishment choices.

Other infections can result from destitute eating as well. Tall blood weight is common, as well as other chronic diseases. Osteoporosis is something that can influence numerous individuals afterward in life since they were not making sound eating choices prior on. You may find yourself enduring from destitute bone wellbeing, hypertension, or indeed heart issues. All of which can be exceptionally requesting on your body and cause major stretch that can ultimately be exceptionally unsafe.

If you need to appear your family simply care almost them, you should begin making choices presently that will assist you to stay in their lives for as long as possible. Poor wellbeing isn't something that as it were influences you. It is additionally something that influences the individuals around you. In the event that they are observing you endure since of poor choices that you simply have made, in a way, that's very selfish. They are enduring as well. Presently, do your best to make the choices that will be the finest not as it were for yourself, but for your family in the long run. This book will appear you how.

CHAPTER 2: UNDERSTANDING YOUR RELATIONSHIP WITH FOOD

Over the course of time, everyone starts to create certain propensities. We create propensities in all fields of our lives. We create cleanliness propensities, nourishment propensities, work propensities, and all sorts of other sorts of propensities. Be that as it may, they are ordinarily lovely unaware to our propensities until they begin to influence us adversely. And indeed at that point, when we start to get it that we are being ineffectively affected by our propensities, it can be exceptionally troublesome to alter them. Since that's what I have it is like.

A propensity is something that we do nearly unknowingly. We are modified to take after these propensities, and it takes a awesome sum of determination to break free from the cycle.

Once you start to get it that your relationship with nourishment has everything to do with the propensities simply have made and propensities that you simply can proceed to shape and develop, at that point it gets to be distant less demanding to alter your mentality.

When you realize the affect and significance of your future and making positive choices approximately these things, it can make you more prepared toward sound eating and less slanted to form choices that contrarily affect you and your future.

To be honest, numerous of us appear to consider long term bleak. We don't see reasons sufficient to alter our propensities since in case we don't accept that we have anything great to look forward to, at that point it doesn't matter whether we make great choices or not. We don't see how ready to really clear our future to be in our best interface. Likely since we don't accept that we have any control over our lives.

If you'll relate to this feeling, don't be frightened. It is very common of the human encounter. We are generally disheartened from taking control and utilizing our control from an early age, and sometimes ceased accepting we have any specialist over our lives since we are ordinarily told what to do by other individuals.

As children, that makes sense. Children don't continuously know what is best for them. But it can energize an awfully defenseless sort of attitude that causes us to have a difficult time understanding that the results of our activities can genuinely start to shape who we are and how we show ourselves to the world.

This is why it is imperative to genuinely take steps to assist you get it yourself and your dietary propensities. When did your propensity start? How did you form that propensity? Why? What benefits do you have got from this propensity? What negative impacts do you have got from this habit?

Ask yourself as numerous of these questions as you possibly can so that you simply start to really have an understanding of how it is merely are forming your future with the nourishment that you are eating. Are you making a sound and energized future, or are you making a future that's bleak and possibly full of negative health consequences?

Next, assess your sense of self teach. Are you competent of keeping up discipline over your choices? Or is this an range where you battle? Teach can be troublesome for everyone, and in case you discover yourself having a difficult time remaining taught, it would do you well to see into diverse ways simply are able to energize yourself to be a more taught individual both in hone and rationally.

Only at that point will you really have what it takes to start a travel of solid eating. Since whether we like it or not, and terrible wellbeing choices are everywhere. They are easy and they are addicting.

If we permit ourselves to be influenced by these poor choices, and do nothing to change our propensities, at that point it doesn't matter whether you eat healthy in some cases or not. The negative impacts will still be grasping your body and holding up to spring up on you once you least expect it.

In a way, unfortunate eating is a self-destructive design that a parcel of us take portion in. Whether typically because of destitute self-esteem, or simply because we are despondent with our circumstances and have no confidence within the future, self-destructive eating designs are unsafe. You've got to look to yourself and truly esteem your life and your future some time recently eating healthy will adhere.

There are numerous ways that you just can do this, and in the event that conceivable, you'll indeed need allude to">to refer to a mental wellbeing proficient for back. In some cases, they can offer assistance us to see predispositions and negative designs in our lives that we stay unaware to. Once those are caught on and acknowledged, at that point it can be that much simpler to overcome them and take the steps that you wish to require in arrange to form positive choices.

Whether you seek out the offer assistance of a qualified proficient or not, there are many things that you can do to alter your mentality. As long as you understand that you just are commendable of a healthy body and a positive future, then you'll permit yourself to require the steps essential to get there.

But if you are doing not feel great almost yourself, it is going to be a parcel harder. By and large, understanding yourself, your propensities, your mental barricades, and your discipline, will assist you in your journey. All of us can take steps each day toward getting to be our best possible selves, and sound eating is one extraordinary step in that direction. And it could be a step able to take today!

CHAPTER 3: THE DANGERS OF DIET TRENDS

Count calories patterns are wild in our society nowadays, and nearly all of them come with perils connected to them. Shockingly, most individuals who are frantic to form cash regularly don't see at the long-term wellbeing results of their items. What they are genuinely concerned approximately is making cash and doing something that will offer assistance them to capitalize off of a desperate desire that numerous individuals need to lose weight in a fast and simple way.

There is something that you just are aiming to need to accept if diet patterns are something that captivate your intrigued. The unfortunate fact of the matter is that there's no sound way to lose weight quick and effortlessly with no work and no healthy eating and no exercise. Losing weight may be a great objective in the event that you're hefty or if you're missing in wellness and you would like additional versatility.

All of us have at times required to begin making way better way of life choices, which is something that we are able do with nourishment and solid body development as restricted to by trusting companies that need to abuse us in arrange to create cash.

Some of the eat less patterns out there are uncommonly unsafe and have critical wellbeing results both long-term and shortterm. Numerous of them depend on strategies that cause us to starve ourselves and Robert body of fundamental supplements. Some of the time, indeed drying out us.

These sorts of eat less patterns are amazingly nauseating. They are taking advantage of individuals who need to be sound but don't know how to go approximately it. They are taking advantage of individuals, regularly ladies in specific, who are disintegrating beneath the weights of unrealistic beauty standards and women who are told that to have any esteem, they must see a certain way.

That is completely unfaithful. Whether you weigh 100 pounds or 700 pounds, you have got esteem. Be that as it may, solid eating is one of the only real ways

that you just are going to be able
to kickstart your digestion system
and give your body with the
nutrients that it needs to work on
its highest possible capacity.

If you're ransacking your body of
the vitamins and minerals that it
needs in arrange to flourish and
trusting a diet trend to instruct you
how to lose weight and have
esteem when all they truly need is
your cash, at that point you're
going to conclusion up advance
behind the line at that point you
were to begin out with. The
terrible truth almost numerous eat
less patterns is that they cause

the body to go into starvation mode.

This can wreck your digestion system and cause you to pick up weight indeed quicker within the future. Don't let yourself be misused by the notices promising simply will lose weight in a quick and simple way. All of that will come with a cost. Not as it were that, but there are wellbeing patterns out there such as the hCG eat less that can really screw up your body and your hormones.

The amusing thing almost eat less patterns is that they often will make it harder for you to lose weight within the future because you are executing undesirable and difficult ways of maintaining your weight. On the off chance that you need to be skinny, don't believe a pill on TV to create you thin. Begin cutting out undesirable sugary and prepared nourishments and supplant them with solid whole-grain wheat and natural natural products and vegetables that will not present chemicals into your body that will make it indeed harder for you to lose weight and that will eventually mess up your body chemistry.

It could seem enticing to be able to lose weight quickly and not have to be sacrifice the negative eating propensities that you have created over your lifetime, but it isn't healthy. You're hurting yourself and preparing your body for further health complications within the future on the off chance that you're not careful about the way you endeavor to lose weight. Make beyond any doubt that you're doing everything in your control to form choices that you simply would need other people to make for themselves.

Do inquire about before you let yourself be swayed by the wind oil sales representative on TV. Look into these things since you're worth doing things the correct way and you deserve a positive future and not one that is complicated by the side impacts of a deals pitch that as it were needs your money and not your wellbeing.

CHAPTER 4: THE FOOD PYRAMID

Most of us have likely seen the nourishment pyramid. Developing up, the nourishment pyramid was regularly utilized as a rule for us to supply us with an thought of how much nourishment and what kind of nourishment we ought to eat every day in arrange to preserve a solid way of life.

Of course, there's continuously prove to state that the nourishment pyramid is adaptable, but overall, on the off chance that you're able to watch the nourishment pyramid you may have a common thought of what is worthy in a sound and nutritious eat less.

While this may in some cases be disputable, it is still great to have a basic food. Conceivably one that you just make yourself. A part of individuals will say that it is now not considered the foremost sound thing to do to eat as numerous grains as the nourishment pyramid may have recommended.

In truth, with later flare-ups of celiac infection, a part of people are touting a no grain way of life as the foremost sound choice.

Rather than depending on the nourishment pyramid for your fundamental rule of what is sound to eat, attempt to require into thought your claim individual encounters with nourishment and go from there. A few individuals are more advantageous with a parcel of grains, and a few are not. Utilize your judgment here to the best of your capacity so that you simply will be able to require steps within the right course for your wellbeing.

The standard nourishment pyramid suggests as takes after:

- Rice, cereal, pasta, and bread, can be as many as 11 servings per day.

- For vegetables and fruits, you ought to have between three and five servings.

- As far as their eggs, you'll have two or three servings every day, given you're not allergic or lactose intolerant.

- When it comes to meet and beans, and other things like nuts and angle or poultry, it is prescribed merely have two or three servings each day.

- Unsurprisingly, things such as sugar and fat and oil are the exceptionally tip of the. Since you ought to not have any of these things in overabundance. Or maybe, utilize them only as vital in order to ensure your most advantageous conceivable way of life.

Again, typically as it were referencing the standard nourishment pyramid. Depending on your claim particular needs and dietary capacities, you may ought to adjust this chart for yourself. But on the off chance that you don't have any specific necessities, usually the standard for the food pyramid that can be utilized to your most prominent conceivable advantage in creating a healthier lifestyle

CHAPTER 5: HOW FOOD CAN BE YOUR MEDICINE

Just as not eating healthily can make you sick, eating healthy foods can often cure illness and alleviate suffering.

 It can also act as a preventive measure against diseases. In fact, an entire healing system called Aryuveda has existed in India for thousands of years.

 This ancient style of healing is used to treat all kinds of ailments simply by changing the diet. Food is literally medicine that has sustained Native Americans for centuries. And it can be applied even today.

 In fact, many remedies are simply healthy foods that have anti-inflammatory properties and the ability to nourish your body from the inside out. Healthy food choices are known to affect everything from infection to cancer.

 And with this ancient healing art, it's never been more obvious.

 Of course, many modern technologies dislike these methods because they have not been scientifically studied, but much of it has been tried and true for thousands of years and will continue to affect the body. Whether you believe in ancient healing arts or not, the fact is that food can ultimately determine whether or not you are susceptible to disease. When you eat well, your body is stronger and can fight off disease and infection much more easily than if you were malnourished following the standard American diet.

 If your body does not have enough vitamins and minerals, it is almost impossible to fight the negative consequences of the disease.
 Sometimes it can even cause diseases. When you eat unhealthy unprocessed foods, certain types of these foods can cause disease and also make you more susceptible to certain types of cancer. Although cancer is still being researched and not fully

understood by the scientific community to truly cure it, there are many cases where people have been able to live long and healthy lives simply by changing their habits. A healthy diet can help reduce the symptoms of many difficult and impossible-to-treat diseases, such as multiple sclerosis.

 As long as you make sure that everything you put into your body is nutritious and provides your organs and cells with all the fuel and resources they need to keep your body strong, they will continue to do so. And they do it to the best of their ability.

However, if you are actively sabotaging your body, they will not be able to fight back as if they were getting enough food. That's why it's so important that you pay attention to how you feed your body. If you don't make active and informed choices about your food, you may regret it.

CHAPTER 6: THE HEALTH BENEFITS OF EATING VEGETABLES

Vegetables are one of the least consumed foods, especially when it comes to the typical American diet. Most people do not understand how important it is to provide the body with vitamins and minerals that only vegetables and fruits can provide. Sometimes people consider vegetables as a way to improve their beauty, but when it comes to improving their health, they become a bit indifferent.

 But now that you're here and reading this book, it's safe to assume that you're ready and able to think about why it's important to eat your vegetables. Here are some of the best reasons to give yourself vegetables as part of your diet every day. First, the body needs fiber to eliminate excess waste. If waste products cannot be found and removed together, they get stuck in the body and can contribute to weight gain and other potential complications.

 Fiber is very important for other reasons as well. It can help you avoid high blood cholesterol and even prevent heart disease, or at least reduce your chances of developing it.

 Folic acid is also found in vegetables, and when you give your body this substance, it can make your red blood cells. It can be very important to prevent anemia and can be very useful, especially for women who tend to need this substance during pregnancy and menstruation.

 Vegetables are also naturally rich in many vitamins, such as vitamins A and C, which help fight infections and keep the body healthy. This can help you speed up the healing process and absorb iron, another way to fight and prevent anemia. Vitamins are high in potassium and this is very useful because it prevents the body from high blood pressure.

Vegetables have been shown to reduce the risk of strokes and other heart-related complications. They can prevent the formation of kidney stones and prevent bone fracture. Eating vegetables is a great way to fight type 2 diabetes and obesity.

Not only that, but it can help you stay strong in your fight against cancer and cancer prevention. Perhaps one of the most redeeming qualities of eating vegetables is that they are very low in fat and certainly not high in calories.

This means you can eat as many vegetables as you want without worrying too much about weight gain. Eating vegetables is a great way to reduce hunger and focus on a healthy lifestyle.

 There are so many good things about vegetables. It is surprising that they are so rare in the American diet. One of the best ways to avoid processed foods with fat, sugar and salt is to get out of the grocery store first.

 Go to the fresh produce section, making conscious choices to provide your body with healthy fresh vegetables instead of buying pasta and other processed foods that are low in truly nutritious vegetables. A healthy diet starts with the body's nutritional choices, and few things are more nutritious than vegetables.

 Due to unhealthy and bad eating habits early in life or even self-imposed, we can often lose our taste for healthy food, but getting back on track is easy. Make time in your life for vegetables. They may take a little longer to prepare, but the benefits are worth it.

CHAPTER 7: THE HEALTH BENEFITS OF EATING FRUITS

It is unfortunate but common knowledge that people who follow the standard American diet do not eat enough fruit. What fruit they eat is usually canned or saturated with sugar. The added sugar and fruit is definitely something that cancels out all the health benefits that eating fruit in its natural state can provide the body.

 Eating too much fruit can cause complications, especially if you have diabetes. Fruits have a lot of natural sugars, and juice gives you a lot of sugar without a lot of fiber, which can give the body excess. The fiber in fruits is one of the things that makes them the healthiest and helps the body reduce heart disease and prevent constipation. Not only that, but high-fiber foods like fruits and vegetables are also very beneficial for weight management because they help you feel full with fewer calories. Not only that, but fruits also contain many vitamins and minerals, especially citrus fruits when it comes to vitamin C.

Vitamin C is a powerhouse when it comes to healing the body, and if you need something to help keep your teeth and gums healthy, vitamin C-rich fruits are sure to help.

Another thing that fruits help the body achieve is the prevention of strokes and kidney stones. Fruits are very useful for supporting the body and preventing and fighting disorders such as skin diseases and heart problems. Fruits can be one of the healthiest ways to help you get extra energy and eliminate the sugar cravings you may experience when trying to eliminate unhealthy foods from your diet.

As long as you don't overdo it with your fruit, like throwing it in a blender and consuming ridiculous amounts of sugar, you can have a healthy snack that satisfies your sweet tooth if you're willing to use it. the enormous power of the fruit.

If you are interested in the health benefits of food, both fruits and vegetables have a natural tendency to help your skin glow and look much more hydrated and nourished. Fruits and vegetables are rich in antioxidants and vitamins and minerals that give your body the hydration it needs to keep your skin and appearance healthy. It can help your hair grow softer and healthier and keep your skin looking youthful. Fruits can even help you stop acne by keeping your body clean of waste products that come through your pores and moisturizing your skin. Fruits are great for keeping your body hydrated due to their high water content and you will quickly start to see the benefits and this aspect.

 Not only that, but fruits are especially good for digestion.

Thanks to its high fiber content, it helps bind waste and helps the body get rid of things that might otherwise cause problems. Therefore, fruits and vegetables can also help you lose weight. Instead of letting the waste products break down and be stored as fat, the body removes them before they reach it.

 Fruits are another great way to fight and prevent disease, even cancer. Certain fruits like apples help keep asthma at bay. Others can significantly lower cholesterol. Grapes, especially red-skinned grapes, are also known to be used in the fight against cancer. They also help fight eye and kidney problems. If you suffer from an infection, the berries are especially helpful. They are rich in antioxidants.

 Just make sure you eat fruits and vegetables that haven't been treated with commercial pesticides because they can absorb these chemicals and make it harder to lose weight and cause problems in the body. You can even eat dried fruits to replace unhealthy and sugary snacks and provide your body with a sweet snack that is quite nutritious. Be aware of the sugar content of dried fruit, as sometimes the added sugars turn this healthy treat into something that will ultimately help you shed pounds.

However, if you eat fruits in a healthy and regular way, fruits can help you lose weight. As long as you haven't eaten too many sweets, the fiber and water content in fruit helps your body feel full and nourishes your cells and organs. The fiber and water content will help you get rid of obesity problems and you will generally feel a huge change in your energy levels. You can use this energy to exercise and work harder to live a healthy lifestyle.

This can be especially effective if you replace sugary junk with healthier fruits, continuing your journey to better health and wellness.

CHAPTER 8: THE BEST MEAT TO EAT FOR HEALTHY LIVING

Meat is usually considered one of the most important staples in email, but you might be surprised to find that some meats are actually healthier than others. Of course we know the difference between red and white meat. Red meat is more often associated with health problems and coronary artery problems, while white meat is generally considered less fatty and healthier.

 Some people may be surprised to learn that there are other things that make muscles unhealthy. Questions like what they are fed while the animals are still alive and the antibiotics and hormones that can be injected into them to make them grow faster or produce more milk, at least in the case of cows. These types of hormones eventually eat away at the flesh and can cause problems in our own bodies. If we are not aware of the choices we make when choosing our foods, they can lead to poor health in the future, including but not limited to cancer and hormonal changes that can be quite debilitating.

 However, if you make sure you get your meat from healthy sources and don't feed the animals extra steroids and antibiotics, you're already ahead of the game. If not, try to research local places where you can get meat that is not spoiled by dangerous industrial standards.

However, even when considering healthy meat choices, some meats are healthier than others. One of the healthiest meats you can eat, especially if you're trying to lose weight, is fish. Fish is lean and full of nutrients. However, you must be careful about the source of the fish.

 Some fish are raised in unhealthy conditions, while others may come from areas that may be contaminated with mercury. Therefore, pregnant women should not eat fish or shellfish. But finding a healthy source of fish can be very beneficial for your body. Fish is rich in omega-3 fatty acids, which help brain function and memory. Overall, Omega 3s are in high demand and the body needs them to function at maximum efficiency, especially in intellectual matters.

 Another great choice is chicken raised in a good environment. Chicken is rich in protein. In fact, it has the highest protein content of any muscle. They are usually raised in good conditions or at least fed a diet that does not cause problems to the human body in the same way that many livestock do.

However, if you eat grass and meat from a reliable supplier, it can also be a great choice. If you're going to eat organic chicken, it's generally less likely that those animals were raised with dangerous carcinogens.

Conventionally raised chickens are usually fed growth-enhancing food, which can cause serious health problems for both the chickens themselves and the people who eat them. They are also given copious amounts of antidepressants and painkillers, sometimes even arsenic and caffeine.

It's dangerous to eat a lot of conventionally raised meat, but if you can find a good supplier, it's definitely worth it.

Turkey is another good meat because it is rich in selenium. It is great for the body, especially because it can help eliminate free radicals and other toxic substances.

However, again, you want to make sure you get your meat from reliable sources, as the norm for conventionally raised chickens and turkeys is that they are treated the same and fed

dangerous chemicals that accelerate their growth and ultimately contaminate humans. bodies with these chemicals.
Eating meat can be very good for your body as long as you don't eat meat that comes from dangerous, conventional farming methods.
The chemicals that these animals often expose us to are very dangerous both for the animals themselves and for the people who consume them. If you want to eat healthy and lose weight, it's better to avoid chemicals that can stay in the body and prevent weight loss.

Even if you don't want to lose weight, eating healthy means avoiding anything that can be dangerous to the body, such as hormones and chemicals that disrupt our delicate systems. Fortunately, there are many sources of healthy meat, whether you want to enjoy poultry, beef or even lamb. There are ways you can grow me healthy and ethical to satisfy your potential desires.

CHAPTER 9: THE DANGERS OF PROCESSED FOODS

It should come as no surprise to anyone that processed food is dangerous. What is surprising, however, is that despite the havoc they wreak on our bodies and minds, they are still allowed on the shelves. Eating unhealthy food is not a personal choice of some people.

 Sometimes, with the way the economy works, poor people have to resort to processed foods because it's a cheap and easy

way to feed a large family on a
shoestring budget.

The hard part is that these foods
end up causing medical problems
that cost even more money than
feeding a large family with healthy,
sustainable options. At the end of
the day, people with little money
seem to suffer though.

Even if you don't have to feed
your family on a shoestring
budget, processed food is just
plain unhealthy. Part of what
makes them addictive is their high
fat and sugar content.

These are often boxed foods that contain pasta and are exceptionally high in sugar. Too much sugar is dangerous in general, but especially for people who are prone to type 2 diabetes. If you consume sugar and in large quantities, you will end up overloading your body and not only will you gain more weight than most likely, but you will also develop health problems.

 Sugar can accelerate the progression of diabetes by causing the development of insulin resistance, which eventually makes it difficult, if not impossible, to control blood sugar.

 Eating too much of these foods, like at every meal or at least every day, will inevitably have a negative effect. Consuming this high amount of fat and sugar regularly can lead to diabetes and obesity, which is common knowledge, as well as heart disease and even cancer. This is extremely dangerous and processed foods should be avoided at all costs. Another danger of eating processed foods is that they are not only addictive, they are highly artificial. Most of the ingredients in these foods do not nourish the body. Rather, they make us feel full, depriving our bodies of vital nutrients needed to function healthily.

 If we eat a crappy diet instead of nutritious food, we end up making fools of ourselves. We don't think right, we don't move right, and we don't act in his highest way. All these things are very harmful and can lead to poor coordination and even depression.

 At some level, we all know that processed foods are not as healthy as the foods we should be eating on a regular basis. Our body knows this, even if our mind is not aware. And we suffer because of it. We are stressed about it. When we eat unhealthy food, whether we are addicted to it or not, our body knows it. And whether it's a subconscious event or not, we often punish ourselves. We know we are doing something wrong. We are shocked and saddened by this, although we are currently dealing with it.

 Processed foods are also rich in artificial dyes that have been shown to be highly carcinogenic. When we eat foods with a solid color, we mainly ingest the color. Would you like to eat hair color? Not quite. But these types of chemicals are used in your food. They stay in your body and don't come out. They lubricate your organs from the inside. They are very dangerous and can cause cancer.

 It is also full of conservatives. Processed food lasts a very long time on the shelf. Longer than is healthy and normal. No typical bottle of milk will last for months. It would run and crash. The same with cheeses and the same with other shelf-stable foods.

 Shelf life is important to businesses because they can make more money if their food stays on the shelf longer. They will do anything, no matter what is healthier than the human body, to make sure they make as much money as possible. Preservatives often contain unhealthy and unnatural chemicals and excessive amounts of salt. Neither is good for the body. Processed foods can cause heart problems and hypertension because these foods contain too much salt. High blood pressure is common in people who live on processed foods, and obesity and heart attacks are the leading killers in North America.

 It has everything to do with the standard American diet. The sad thing is, even though you know it's unhealthy, the chemicals and high sugar and fat content make these processed foods highly addictive.

 The body begins to crave them and this can be almost as dangerous as drug addiction. Depending on food that is neither nutritious nor healthy can have long-term consequences for your health and development.

 Another way processed foods contribute to obesity is that we digest them too quickly compared to healthy, fiber-rich foods. If we digest these foods quickly and they don't fill us up because we don't get the fiber that makes us feel full, we don't even expend as much energy as if we were digesting healthy foods.

 This means that we eat more and digest less, which leads to rapid and rapid weight gain. If you follow a diet high in processed foods, your body will burn a lot more calories. You'll burn a lot more calories when you eat healthy, whole foods that are high in fiber.

 Unfortunately, this means that people who live and thrive on a diet of processed foods end up gaining weight whether they want

to or not. And they don't give you as much energy because they're not nutritious. You will probably feel tired, lethargic and over full because you are eating a lot more of these unhealthy sugary foods without feeling full or satisfied.
 Processed food does not metabolize properly in our body. They quickly become fat. Not only that, but they have a lot of fat. They are often full of hidden fats and sugars. Vegetable oil is one of the main ingredients in many of these processed foods, along with high fructose corn syrup, which is a huge culprit in weight gain.

If all the processed foods on the shelves contained high fructose corn syrup, and most do, it's no wonder North America is facing the worst obesity epidemic in the history of the world. Hydrogenated oils are very unhealthy because they do not break down.

They stay in your body and combine with fat cells. These oils make it much more difficult to burn fat. They are more difficult to get rid of and this type of stubborn fat can lead to obesity very quickly. Processed food ingredients lack most of the nutritional value that humans need to function at their best. We need the fiber and vitamins and minerals found in real food before we can truly thrive.

 If you find that you can't avoid processed foods completely, you should at least eat them in moderation. They are dangerous. They can make us lethargic, irritable and generally unhappy.

 Our attitudes can change from positive to negative when we abandon a healthy diet and end up eating only processed foods that are too sweet, too fatty and unhealthy.

Our body needs food. The easiest and most beneficial thing you can do for yourself is to provide your body with this nutrition. Changing routines, such as living on processed foods, can be hard to get used to and can be very frustrating at times.

You need to spend a lot more time in the kitchen cooking and considering your health and nutrition. But in the end, eating processed food can kill you and tear you apart. In fact, you are consuming toxins and avoiding foods that can act as antioxidants, giving you a chance to rid your body of waste.

Processed foods are the same as junk food. They are no different. They are healthier than junk food. These are snacks in disguise. To get healthy and feel healthy, avoiding processed foods at all costs is the first and most effective step you can take. Don't be fooled by the packaging that claims these foods are healthy. They are saturated and fat and sugar and salt and have nothing to nourish your body. Do what you can to change the way you rely on processed foods. Healthy eating is easy and possible if you can afford it.

Just remember the strategy of walking through the grocery store to pick up fresh produce and meats instead of walking down aisles full of dangerous and tempting packaging that hides the dangers of processed foods.

CHAPTER 10: BRINGING IT ALL TOGETHER WITH MEAL PLANNING

Meal planning can be one of the most important aspects of developing a healthy lifestyle. When we can't imagine the future of our eating, it can be very easy to give in to the unhealthy food we've become addicted to. Especially when we tend to eat them instead of eating the food that nourishes us.

 Meal planning is quite a job. This can be a little scary, especially for those who suffer from disorganization. If you have trouble planning your meals, don't worry. Whether you're creative in the kitchen or not, there are lots of fun and easy ways to get started with meal planning.

 You can buy many meal plan packages. Many of them have the ability to order cooking boxes full of fresh food and contain recipes that you can use. This can be very useful if you are not used to cooking, which is often the case. Especially when bad eating habits and a busy work schedule make it difficult to find time for healthy and nutritious meals. The first step in meal planning is research. If you are going to recover, you need to look at your options.

 Researching recipes is the best place to start. Collecting a binder full of healthy foods you want to try can be both fun and educational. It will open your mind to different foods that you may have looked down on or teach you about things you didn't know before.

 Recipes can be very wonderful. Especially if you are interested in new discoveries. Cooking can be hard to learn, but once you get the hang of it, you'll be surprised how much freedom you have to create healthy and delicious meals!

 Check out recipe books and magazines and get a collection of recipes you want to try. Start with the things that seem the most delicious and nutritious, and if you're new to the kitchen, you can also go for the things that seem the easiest. Next, you need to organize your recipes in a simple way that is easy to navigate. If you feel overwhelmed by the lack of organization, it makes meal planning much more difficult.

 When starting a new habit, you want to make sure everything is as easy as possible. Too many changes at once can stress your system, and you should always try to make small, simple changes until they become a new habit.

 Make sure they are readily available so you can start cooking easily. If you use a binder, you should consider laminating the sides or using plastic sleeves to prevent them from being affected by water or other food contamination when they are used in the kitchen.

 When organizing recipes, it would help to organize them by breakfast, lunch, dinner and snacks. This makes it easy to find the right recipes when you start cooking. If you want, you can even organize the folder by days of the week and plan meals for each day and print the folder that way.

There are many ways to organize your recipes. Intuitively do what makes the most sense to you. Don't force yourself to join an organization that doesn't work for you. Instead, do what works best for you in your life.

 Be sure to take the time to regularly search for new recipes that stand out to you to keep the creative juices flowing and your kitchen exciting. You can try many different recipes and the more you try, the more interesting your healthy eating journey will be!

 Next, you should look at software like Microsoft Office Excel to help you organize your meal planning. Excel has many templates to choose from to help you plan your meals by day, time of day and week. This can be a very valuable resource!

 If you don't want to use Excel, you can also download apps to your phone, tablet, or other device to help you make better use of your time and resources.

You can even go the old fashioned route and buy a laptop designed specifically for meal planning. This is an important step in ensuring that meals are organized and easily accessible.

Making a meal plan is very helpful in your healthy eating journey. Building good habits takes time and patience, and it's inevitable that you'll slip up somewhere along the way.

But that doesn't mean you have to stay stuck! In fact, it just means that you have to pick yourself up and keep trying, because giving up is a lot easier than sticking to your plans. One thing that can really help with meal planning is keeping a theme. For example, many people have certain themes, such as Taco Tuesday or some other day reserved for a certain type of food. If you think it would help you stay on track, copy this type of meal planning. This is done for a reason as it works and helps keep things simple and smooth.

 It can be very tedious to have to do a lot of planning and preparation every week or month, so if you want to keep things simple, this can be a good way to do it. You could have a bi-weekly food theme, say Taco Tuesday one night and maybe Rice and Veggie Tuesday the next night, and alternate between them. There is no wrong way to plan your meals. You must follow.

Without tracking, everything else becomes unnecessary and complicated. Something that can really help you succeed in meal planning is accountability. If you tell someone who knows and cares about you that you are trying to plan your meals, ask them if they would be willing to help you stick to your routine.

They can help you by asking questions about how things are going and whether or not you are staying on track. They may also want to encourage and encourage you in your endeavors.

However they support you, they can be very rewarding for both of you. If they are positive and encouraging people, it can be good to know that you have people in your corner who really want you to succeed. Just make sure you remove toxic people who bring you down, draw attention to you, or make you feel like you're struggling to reach your goals.

Of course, constructive feedback can be very helpful, but if you don't seek out constructive feedback, it can sometimes be toxic. Make sure you understand the difference between a toxic person masquerading as a supportive person and a supportive person who really wants you to succeed.

 Another way to take responsibility is to take personal responsibility. Personal responsibility can be achieved through journalism and self-insurance. Talking to yourself about your goals and what you are doing internally or out loud can be a good way to help you focus and ask yourself if you are doing the things you hope to achieve.

  If you find that you don't, instead of beating yourself up, reflect on your barriers and move forward as you begin to uncover them. The only way to fail is if you don't try. If you try, everything will end up in place because you put in the effort and create positive changes in your life.

  Journaling is useful for many reasons. You can use them to record what you ate, when and how much. This will give you a good idea of what you can realistically expect from yourself. Things you are not happy with should be addressed and considered. But instead of being mad at yourself for not being picky right away, remember that this is a process and you have to take it slow.

 Instead of completely changing your routine and planning every meal for the next month even though you've never done it before, instead start slowly by simplifying one or two meals a week and then gradually adding the rest as you feel comfortable. with the process. Make it something that won't shock your system. Gradual change is the most sustainable. And keeping a journal of your experiences will help you uncover your inner thoughts about the process and the things you may not have even known were holding you back.

 You will begin to perceive patterns in your behavior and perhaps predict when you might be tempted to deviate from your path and why. If you can identify these trigger points, it will be easier to avoid them in the future. Meal planning can be a lot of fun and exciting. Even if you are not the type to enjoy this type of organization, it can be very useful to think about what you are putting in your body and take the necessary steps. Everyone deserves the chance to become

the healthiest, healthiest version
of themselves, and with meal
planning and a healthy dose of
self-esteem, you'll be on your
way to healthy eating.

CONCLUSION

Starting a healthy diet can be very
difficult, especially if you haven't
been able to develop healthy
eating habits since you were
young. However, it is not
impossible to become a healthier
and more active person.

Fortunately, we wake up alive
every day and breathing is the day
we can begin to heal ourselves
and move forward in life.

Becoming the best version of
yourself can seem scary at first,
but when you realize that every
choice you make affects your life,
whether positive or negative, it
becomes much easier to see the
course of your actions before they
come back to haunt you. haunt us
. . Bad eating habits are definitely
choices that come back to haunt
us. If we're not careful, we start
developing health problems later
in life because we didn't know

what we were putting in our bodies when we were younger. Eating healthy and exercising is the only way to create a healthy and happy body and mind.

 We become crazy and anxious when we are stuck in our houses all day, eating only processed foods high in sugar and fat, and sitting around watching TV without exercise. The standard American diet is dangerous and costs people their lives. Don't let yourself become one of those people. Instead, make the choices you need to make to truly improve yourself and become the best version of you possible. Make choices that will make your family proud and give them your presence in their lives for years to come.

 If we don't take care of ourselves, it's actually very selfish. We are surrounded by people who care deeply about who we are and the value we bring to their lives, whether we realize it or not. Everyone deserves the opportunity to take control of their future and create positive change that will benefit them for years to come. Healthy eating is just one of the many ways to heal yourself and prepare your mind and body for the future. If you want to be independent and active for as long as possible without racking up thousands and thousands of dollars in medical bills and other expenses, eating healthy is something you should start sooner rather than later.

 If not, it will inevitably become your life both materially and physically. By reading this book and using the information it contains, you are now better prepared to take the first step towards a healthy lifestyle.

Planning your meals and raising awareness of why it's important to make healthy food choices will greatly improve your quality of life now and years from now. All you have to do is stick to it and you'll start seeing the positive health effects of a healthy diet right away! All you have to do is try. You can do it!